The Sheldon Short Guide to
Asthma

Mark Greener spent a decade in biomedical research before joining *MIMS Magazine* for GPs in 1989. Since then, he has written on health and biology for magazines worldwide for patients, healthcare professionals and scientists. He is a member of the Royal Society of Biology and is the author of 21 other books, including *The Heart Attack Survival Guide* (2012) and *The Holistic Health Handbook* (2013), both published by Sheldon Press. Mark lives with his wife, three children and two cats in a Cambridgeshire village.

GW00775753

Sheldon Short Guides

A list of titles in the Overcoming Common Problems series
is also available from Sheldon Press, 36 Causton Street,
London SW1P 4ST and on our website at
www.sheldonpress.co.uk

Asthma
Mark Greener

Depression
Dr Tim Cantopher

Diabetes
Mark Greener and Christine
Craggs-Hinton

Heart Attacks
Mark Greener

Liver Disease
Mark Greener

Memory Problems
Dr Sallie Baxendale

Phobias and Panic
Professor Kevin Gournay

Stroke Recovery
Mark Greener

Worry and Anxiety
Dr Frank Tallis

THE SHELDON SHORT GUIDE TO
ASTHMA

Mark Greener

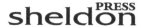

First published in Great Britain in 2016

Sheldon Press
36 Causton Street
London SW1P 4ST
www.sheldonpress.co.uk

British Library Cataloguing-in-Publication Data
A catalogue record for this book is available from the
British Library

ISBN 978-1-84709-380-6
eBook ISBN 978-1-84709-381-3

Typeset by Fakenham Prepress Solutions, Fakenham,
Norfolk NR21 8NN
First printed in Great Britain by Ashford Colour Press
Subsequently digitally reprinted in Great Britain

eBook by Fakenham Prepress Solutions, Fakenham,
Norfolk NR21 8NN

Produced on paper from sustainable forests

To Yasmin, Rory, Ophelia and Rose, with love

Contents

A note to the reader   ix

A note on references   x

Introduction   xi

1   What is asthma?   1

2   Asthma – types and triggers   8

3   Diagnosing asthma   25

4   Treating asthma in adults   31

5   Beyond drugs   48

A note to the reader

This is not a medical book and is not intended to replace advice from your doctor. Consult your pharmacist or doctor if you believe you have any of the symptoms described, and if you think you might need medical help.

A note on references

I used numerous medical and scientific studies to write the book that this Sheldon Short is based on: *Coping with Asthma in Adults*. Unfortunately, there isn't space to include references in this short summary. You can find these in *Coping with Asthma in Adults*, which also discusses the issues in more detail. I have updated some facts and figures.

Introduction

Asthma often evokes images of wheezing children puffing on inhalers. However, around four in every five asthma sufferers are adults. Some have lived with asthma since childhood. In some, symptoms faded during adolescence, but later resurfaced. Some develop asthma for the first time as adults: work-related factors may cause up to a quarter of asthma cases in adults, for instance.

Modern drugs mean that deaths from asthma are, thankfully, now rare. Nevertheless, around 1,200 people die every year from asthma in the UK, the overwhelming majority of whom are adults. Better care could prevent up to 90 per cent of deaths and 75 per cent of hospital admissions due to asthma. In addition, poorly managed asthma undermines almost every aspect of life, from sleep to social life to sex.

Yet asthma in adults rarely receives the attention it deserves. For instance, allergies – the 'classic' cause of asthma in children – underlie, at most, only half of cases in adults. And at least half of people aged 65 years and over have three or more diseases. Some of these other diseases complicate asthma's diagnosis and management. Nevertheless, relatively few studies examine asthma caused by factors other than allergy or the underlying biology in adults, which is essential to develop new treatments. Indeed, many studies exclude older patients or those with other diseases. This simplifies analysis and may protect volunteers from side effects. But such exclusions make it difficult for doctors to extrapolate from the study to the adults in their clinic.

Such issues help explain why asthma in adults often remains poorly managed. In one large international study that included the UK, called INSPIRE, adults with asthma experienced, on average, one attack (exacerbation) every month. About a quarter of exacerbations were severe. Even people reporting supposedly well-controlled asthma experienced, on average, just over six exacerbations annually.

This Sheldon Short focuses on adults living with asthma. (We'll not cover asthma in pregnancy and breastfeeding, which are discussed in the original book. Please speak to your doctor or midwife.) We'll consider diagnosis and triggers as well as the drugs and other approaches adults can take to control their symptoms, enrich their quality of life and perform the activities of daily life that everyone else takes for granted.

1

What is asthma?

According to Asthma UK (<www.asthma.org.uk>), doctors and nurses treat around 4.3 million adults for asthma. Yet asthma in adults often remains undiagnosed. For instance, older people may mistakenly regard breathlessness or wheeze as part of growing older. However, breathlessness and wheeze are often signs of asthma, chronic obstructive pulmonary disease (COPD) or another disease. So, get yourself checked.

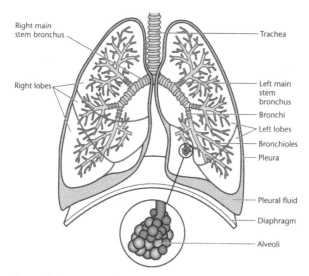

Figure 1 Anatomy of the lungs

Inside our lungs

At rest, a healthy person typically breathes 12 to 20 times each minute, inhaling and exhaling around 500 ml of air. Our lungs don't expand fully each time we take a breath. Most adults can expel between 3 and 5 litres of air after taking the deepest breath they can.

Your left lung, which has two lobes, lies over your heart. Your right lung is slightly larger and has three lobes. Your ribcage surrounds and protects the spongy, fragile lungs and anchors some of the muscles you use to breathe (Figure 1).

Muscles and breathing

Usually, you rely on two sets of muscles to breathe.

- The diaphragm is a thick sheet of muscle under the lungs, anchored to the ribcage, the sternum (breastbone) and the spine.
- The intercostal muscles run between each rib.

When relaxed, the diaphragm is dome-shaped. When you inhale, your diaphragm flattens, and the intercostals contract. This pulls the ribcage up and out, which increases the space in the chest. Air flows through your mouth and nose, along your windpipe (trachea) and into your lungs. The diaphragm and intercostals then relax and the chest 'springs' back to its original shape. This expels the air, now rich in carbon dioxide. Other muscles aid breathing, such as when you exercise.

From the nose to the alveoli

Air flows from the mouth and nose along the trachea. Horseshoe-shaped rings of cartilage – rather like the rings on a vacuum cleaner hose – protect the trachea from crushing.

The trachea forks into two major bronchi, one to each lung. Each major bronchus divides another 10 to 25 times into bronchi and then bronchioles, ending in between 300 million and 500 million alveoli, which look like tiny cauliflower florets (Figure 2). This shape packs a vast area into a relatively small volume:

- Our lungs contain approximately 1,500 miles of airways.
- The surface area of an adult's alveoli is about 70 m^2 – roughly the same as a tennis court.
- A network of around 620 miles of capillaries – small, thin blood vessels – surrounds the alveoli (Figure 2).

Oxygen dissolves in the fluid covering the alveoli and crosses into the blood. Red blood cells pick up and

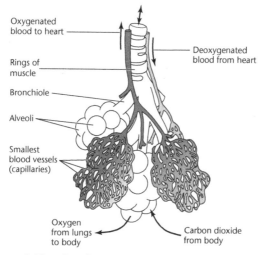

Oxygenated blood to heart

Deoxygenated blood from heart

Rings of muscle

Bronchiole

Alveoli

Smallest blood vessels (capillaries)

Oxygen from lungs to body

Carbon dioxide from body

Figure 2 The alveoli

carry oxygen to your tissues. Red blood cells transport some 'waste' carbon dioxide back to the lungs. About 90 per cent of the carbon dioxide reaches the lungs dissolved in blood.

Age-related changes in breathing

Almost every organ in your body, including your airways, changes as you age. For example:

- Your voice may become quieter, slightly hoarse and 'weaker'. With age, voice usually deepens in women and rises in men.
- After your mid-20s, the number of alveoli declines, reducing the area for gas exchange. Environmental factors – especially smoking – can speed alveoli destruction.
- Your diaphragm, intercostals and other muscles weaken.
- Your chest and lungs become less elastic. So, you drive air from your lungs with less force as you age.

Normally, we have more lung function than we need to perform our daily activities. Nevertheless, age-related changes help explain why asthma can pose a particular problem for adults – they have less in reserve.

Symptoms of asthma

In allergic asthma, an allergen (allergy trigger) inflames the tissues lining the lungs. The swollen tissues narrow the airways, which reduces airflow. As the inflammation increases, the airway becomes narrower and the symptoms worsen (Figure 3 overleaf).

Asthmatic airways are 'twitchy' (hyper-responsive): they narrow (bronchoconstrict) excessively

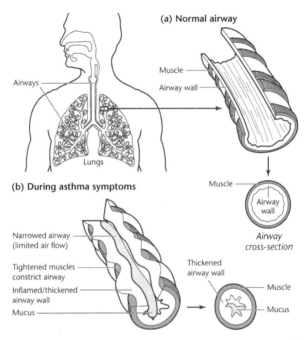

Figure 3 Normal (a) and asthmatic (b) airways

when exposed to, for example, cold air, fog, perfume, some chemicals at work and tobacco smoke. Bronchoconstriction helps keep potentially harmful substances away from the delicate lung lining. However, in people with asthma this narrowing can trigger an attack. In many adults, asthma seems to arise without an allergic reaction.

No two asthma patients show exactly the same pattern of symptoms. Asthma severity and the frequency of attacks often vary over time in the same person. Essentially, however, during asthma attacks,

When to seek urgent medical help

Never underestimate an asthma attack. During some severe asthma attacks, the airways become completely blocked and the person can suffocate. Phone 999 immediately if you have any of the following:

- You feel your bronchodilator (reliever) is not really helping your symptoms.
- You experience severe and constant wheeze, cough or chest tightness. Wheeze may be especially loud. But people with very severe asthma, when there is insufficient airflow, may not wheeze.
- You are too breathless to speak, or talk in words rather than sentences.
- Your pulse is racing.
- You feel agitated or restless.
- You feel drowsy, confused or exhausted.
- Your lips or fingernails look blue.
- Some people hunch forward during a severe attack.

Try not to panic. Deaths from asthma are rare, especially with prompt treatment. Furthermore, severe asthma attacks usually (but not always) develop over 6 to 48 hours. So, remain alert to changes in your symptoms, regularly measuring your peak flow (page 26) and agree a self-management plan with your doctor or asthma nurse. Your partner, carer or colleagues should know how to recognize a severe attack and when to call 999.

the narrowing limits airflow and so hinders oxygen and carbon dioxide exchange. This causes symptoms including:

- cough, which may be the main or only symptom in mild asthma;
- wheeze: a whistling, sighing sound, which tends to be worse in the morning (when the airways are naturally narrower), during exercise or in cold air;
- shortness of, or gasping for, breath. Night-time breathlessness, in particular, indicates poorly controlled asthma (page 11);
- chest tightness, which some people describe as a band around or a weight on their chest.

Initially, the obstruction is largely reversible as the attack abates or with treatment. However, chronic (long-lasting) inflammation thickens and scars the airway walls. These and other changes – called 'remodelling' – can permanently and irreversibly reduce airway diameter, which makes a severe attack more likely. The more severe and long-lasting the asthma, the worse this remodelling becomes.

2

Asthma – types and triggers

Asthma is an umbrella term, covering various patterns of symptoms and a multitude of causes. To optimize your treatment, discuss your symptoms and triggers with your doctor or nurse. You could keep a diary recording your symptoms and what you were doing.

Allergic asthma

Asthma can arise from an allergy to pollen, house dust mite, animal dander (dead skin and hair) and so on. Some doctors suggest regarding asthma that emerges before the age of 30 years as allergic until proven otherwise.

In people with allergic asthma, an 'allergen' inappropriately triggers the immune defences that the body usually uses to recognize and eradicate invading parasites. This causes inflamed, swollen lung tissues.

Unfortunately, we're surrounded by potential allergens:

- *Pollen* You don't need to live next to a meadow or wood to suffer pollen-triggered asthma. Scientists found ragweed pollen 400 miles out to sea and 2 miles up in the atmosphere. Grass pollen deposits within 3 metres of the parent plant. But grass is everywhere, even in the centre of towns and cities.
- *Fungi* Several fungal species can trigger asthma. For example, *Cladosporium* and *Alternaria* grow on dead

organic material (such as decaying leaves). Levels of spores from these fungi peak around harvest time.

- *Mould* The dark stain at the corner of a window where water collects or in the bathroom of a poorly ventilated house could be a mould (a type of fungus) such as *Aspergillus* or *Penicillium*, which can trigger asthma.

- *House dust mite* Beds, soft toys and carpets are home to millions of these microscopic creatures that feed mainly on dead skin cells. A gram of house dust may contain up to 5,000 mites. A typical bed mattress contains about two million mites, which use enzymes to digest dead skin. The enzymes accumulate in the mites' faeces. When inhaled, the enzymes can trigger asthma.

- *Animal dander, feathers and urine* In addition to pets, many people work with animals, in food production, laboratories, zoos, shops and so on. Allergies caused by cats and dogs tend to worsen during the winter, when the house is less well ventilated and pets spend more time indoors.

Intrinsic asthma

In many adults, asthma seems to arise without an allergic reaction. This 'intrinsic' asthma usually emerges in people aged between 40 and 50 years. Doctors may consider asthma that emerges after the age of 40 years as intrinsic until proven otherwise.

Severe asthma

In 5 to 10 per cent of asthmatics, symptoms remain poorly controlled despite standard drugs – so-called severe asthma. Patients may develop:

- severe symptoms almost continually;
- 'brittle asthma': intermittent severe attacks, with normal lung function and no marked symptoms in between;
- mild asthma that occasionally flares into a severe attack.

Several factors can contribute to severe asthma:

- Continual or repeated exposure to an allergen.
- Remodelling may mean that the airway is permanently narrowed.
- Respiratory infections may trigger severe asthma in susceptible people.
- About 80 per cent of people with severe asthma have experienced inflamed sinuses. It's not clear whether sinusitis causes severe asthma, whether sinusitis and asthma arise from the same underlying inflammation, or both.
- Smoking increases the frequency and severity of symptoms and exacerbations, and hastens the decline in lung function.
- Around three-quarters of people with severe asthma are overweight or obese.

The treatment plan depends on your pattern of symptoms and your risk factors.

Recalcitrant asthma

'Recalcitrant asthma' refers to symptoms that do not respond adequately to treatment. Many people with recalcitrant asthma suffer severe symptoms. But mild symptoms might not respond fully to treatment.

Recalcitrant asthma arises from several causes:

- Misdiagnosis: several diseases – such as COPD, congestive heart failure and vocal cord dysfunction – can mimic asthma's symptoms. If your asthma treatment doesn't seem to be working, ask your doctor or nurse to investigate other possible causes.
- Inadequate control of a trigger, such as allergens, smoking or sinusitis, can mean the treatment does not work as well as it should.
- Doctors and asthma nurses don't always treat asthma aggressively enough, possibly because they worry about side effects.
- Patients fail to take their medication properly (poor adherence – page 23).
- Remodelling can lead to the obstruction becoming 'fixed' and less responsive.
- The inflammation may be too severe for inhaled steroids ('preventer') to tackle effectively.
- Some people 'naturally' show impaired responses to steroids.

Changing treatments often helps. So, speak to your doctor or asthma nurse.

Nocturnal asthma: a wake-up call

Around 60 per cent of people with asthma find that their symptoms are worse at night and in the early morning. Three main changes contribute to this 'nocturnal asthma':

- In healthy people, airway diameter and lung function peak around 4 p.m. and reach a minimum around 4 a.m. The difference between peak and trough lung function is much greater in asthma patients.

- Inflammation seems to worsen during the night in people with nocturnal asthma more than in people with asthma of similar severity who do not wake.
- Many people with asthma experience their most severe chest tightness and wheezing when they get up in the morning. This seems to reflect the combination of narrow bronchi, increased physical activity and worse inflammation.

Nocturnal asthma remains under-diagnosed, partly because some asthmatics feel that disturbed nights are inevitable or part of ageing. Nevertheless, waking at night wheezing or breathless is one of the strongest indicators that your asthma is poorly controlled. You should see your doctor or asthma nurse.

Exercise-induced asthma

Exercise triggers symptoms in 80 to 90 per cent of people with asthma. Some people experience asthma symptoms only when they exercise. But these symptoms are not an excuse to become a couch potato: a third of elite athletes show exercise-induced bronchoconstriction.

When you exercise, your muscles demand more oxygen. In response, your respiration rate rises and your airways open. In healthy people, bronchi remain open throughout exercise. In people with exercise-induced asthma, the drier and cooler air triggers the hypersensitive bronchi to narrow, causing one or more of the following:

- You experience shortness of breath or chest tightness 5–15 minutes after starting to work out.
- Your endurance unexpectedly declines or doesn't improve when you increase your workout intensity.

- You cough or wheeze 5–15 minutes after starting to work out.

Symptoms during the first five minutes of a workout do not usually indicate exercise-induced asthma but may suggest poorly controlled asthma, poor fitness or injury to the chest muscles. The following tips may help:

- Improve your physical fitness. As fitness improves, you use less of your lungs' capacity at any particular level of activity. Fitness also reduces air's cooling and drying effect.
- Warm up for at least ten minutes before exercising.
- Cover your mouth and nose with a scarf or mask in cold weather. If possible, exercise in a warm environment with humidified air.
- Avoid allergens and pollution (page 22) – don't jog through the woods or fields, or exercise in front of an open window on a polluted city street.
- At the end of exercise, cool down or gradually reduce the exercise intensity.
- Wait at least two hours after eating before exercising.
- Choose the right exercise. Running is more likely to trigger asthma than cycling. Both are more likely to induce asthma than swimming. If cold air is a trigger, avoid winter sports.
- Take a short-acting bronchodilator (page 42) 15 minutes before and, if needed, during exercise. Keep your inhaler close by, such as on the touchline or by the side of the pool.
- Sodium cromoglicate and nedocromil (page 39) prevent exercise-induced symptoms in between 70 and 85 per cent of patients.

Drug-induced asthma

Several medicines can trigger or exacerbate asthma. Aspirin, for example, may precipitate an attack in up to a fifth of people with asthma. So, don't use aspirin or related medicines called non-steroidal anti-inflammatory drugs (NSAIDs; e.g. ibuprofen, naproxen and diclofenac) as tablets, creams, gels, even those bought without a prescription, without speaking to a doctor, pharmacist or nurse.

Beta-blockers treat, among other conditions, dangerously high blood pressure, some anxiety symptoms and glaucoma (page 38). Beta-blockers cause airways to narrow; this isn't usually enough to cause respiratory symptoms in non-asthmatics, but the constriction can provoke an attack in people with asthma. Enough beta-blocker can reach the bloodstream from eye drops used to treat glaucoma to trigger asthma. Doctors can usually find an alternative.

Be careful of herbal medicines

Many plants contain salicylates, which are chemically related to aspirin. So, make sure that the herbalist knows you suffer from asthma (even if you're not consulting for respiratory symptoms). Likewise, your doctor, nurse and pharmacist should know if you're taking herbal treatments.

Food additives and asthma

Many people believe that food allergies cause or contribute to their asthma. However, only 1 in every 500 to 10,000 adults is truly allergic to food. Nevertheless, food manufacturers may use salicylates as preservatives in, for example, hot dogs, ice cream, sandwich spreads and soft drinks. A wide range of other preservatives, colours and antioxidants can trigger asthma in sensitive people. For example, the yellow dye tartrazine triggers symptoms in around half of people with aspirin-sensitive asthma. So, read the label.

If you feel that food causes or exacerbates your asthma, speak to your GP or nurse. You could keep a diary to see if a pattern emerges. If a food may contribute to your asthma, a dietician will help you exclude it from your diet to see if your asthma improves. You may also undergo a 'challenge' test (page 29) to see if the food triggers symptoms. Don't be tempted to exclude the food from your diet yourself – you could cut out important nutrients.

Occupational asthma

At least 350 agents may trigger occupational asthma. Indeed, work-related factors probably cause between a tenth and a quarter of asthma cases among adults. However, doctors may have diagnosed only a third of occupational asthma cases.

Broadly, occupational factors can trigger asthma in three ways:

- Certain allergens can, over time, sensitize the immune system. Exposure to very low levels of the trigger can then provoke symptoms. Asthma caused by occupational allergens tends to emerge several months or even years after exposure starts.
- Chemicals can irritate the lung lining, damaging the airways and exacerbating inflammation. A single exposure to high levels (e.g. from a fire or chemical spill) of some airway irritants can cause 'non-allergic' occupational asthma within minutes

or hours. Frequent lower-intensity exposures to certain chemicals may also induce asthma.

- Various non-specific factors – such as dust, cold air and physical exercise – can provoke pre-existing asthma or undermine lung function.

Almost everyone is exposed to potential asthma triggers at work – some printers produce ozone (a form of pollution), for example. Nevertheless, certain occupations are at especially high risk:

- Bakers can develop asthma triggered by, for instance: flours; alpha-amylase (an enzyme that helps yeast work); contaminants such as mites and fungi; and lupin products, sometimes used to manufacture bread, pasta, pastries and soups.
- Enzymes handled by, for example, detergent manufacturers, research staff and healthcare professionals can evoke allergic reactions. Kitchen staff using papain to tenderize meat can develop respiratory symptoms.
- Numerous chemicals can trigger asthma, including diisocyanates in certain paints, inks and adhesives.
- Wood dust can trigger asthma.
- Dander, urine and blood can provoke asthma among people working with animals.
- Latex used in, for example, adhesives, foam, carpet backings, medical gloves, catheters, condoms and balloons can provoke asthma. People sensitive to natural rubber latex may cross-react to certain foods and plants, including avocados, bananas and the weeping fig.
- Colophony solder flux can be another trigger. Soldering releases a fume of acids and other chemicals that can trigger asthma.
- Pollen and spider mites – a pest affecting various

crops grown in greenhouses and fruit orchards – can trigger asthma in horticulture workers.

If you suffer asthma at work but symptoms are absent or less severe after work, at weekends or on holiday, you may suffer from occupational asthma. Asthmatic symptoms can, however, occur several hours after exposure to the trigger. Furthermore, on repeated exposure, people with occupational asthma take longer to recover. So, symptoms may not improve over the weekend, but abate only after you've been on holiday. To complicate matters further, non-specific triggers can cause symptoms at home, even if the cause is work-based. This can make diagnosing work-related asthma difficult.

Infective asthma

Viruses may contribute to 80 per cent of asthma exacerbations. So, monitor your peak flow especially carefully during lung infections and follow your self-management plan.

Influenza isn't just a bad cold. Flu is potentially fatal, especially for people with chronic respiratory diseases (including severe asthma) and certain other ailments. During the 2014–15 season, which wasn't an epidemic year, flu caused 16,415 extra deaths in England and Wales. That's more than the death toll from breast (11,716 in 2012) or prostate (10,837) cancer. Older people are also more likely to suffer serious complications – such as bronchitis or pneumonia – if they contract flu. So, get your flu jab. Doctors may also advocate pneumococcal vaccine for people with asthma, to protect against pneumonia and other serious diseases.

Sex

In some people with asthma, emotional excitement or physical exertion during sex can trigger an attack. Using a bronchodilator before sex may help prevent you becoming breathless for the wrong reasons.

Occasionally, highly sensitive people suffer an attack if they kiss someone who has consumed a food or medicine that triggers their exacerbations. A few people are allergic to chemicals in spermicides, lubricants, latex (used in some condoms) or semen. So, inform your partner of any drugs or foods that exacerbate your asthma.

Diseases that affect asthma control

Asthma is common. So, many people suffer from other ailments, some of which may undermine asthma control, including:

- Arthritis, weaknesses due to nerve or muscle problems, or some other physical impairments may make using inhalers difficult. Discuss changing the inhaler, using an aid or oral medications with your doctor, nurse or pharmacist.
- Some medicines (page 14) or devices (e.g. made of latex) used to treat concurrent disease can exacerbate asthma. Doctors can usually find an alternative.
- Some diseases directly increase the risk of developing asthma or suffering an exacerbation. The following sections of this chapter look at some common examples.

Hay fever

The respiratory tract is continuous, so inflammation in the nose can spread to the lungs (or vice versa).

Indeed, up to 75 per cent of people with asthma have rhinitis (an allergen triggers inflammation inside your nose). So, treating rhinitis with steroid nasal sprays can improve asthma and vice versa. If you suffer from hay fever (allergic rhinitis) or perennial rhinitis (non-seasonal symptoms caused by, for example, animals or house dust mites) ask your nurse or GP to help you optimize treatment of both conditions.

Chronic sinusitis and polyps

Sinuses are small cavities behind your cheekbones, eyes and forehead, and on either side of the bridge of your nose. Sinuses open into your nasal airways and help control the air's temperature and water content. Sinusitis occurs when the sinuses become inflamed and swollen, often during an infection or following exposure to aller-gens or irritants, such as air pollution, tobacco smoke, pesticides, disinfectants and household detergents.

Mucus produced by your sinuses drains into your nose through small channels. Infections and inflam-mation can block these channels. So, mucus fills the sinus, causing:

- pain
- tender areas
- a blocked or runny nose
- in some cases, a fever.

Chronic sinusitis, which lasts more than 12 weeks, increases an adult's risk of developing asthma.

Tissues lining the sinuses can swell and expand into the nose, forming a polyp (Figure 4 overleaf), which hinders nasal breathing, impairs smell and may increase asthma risk. Indeed, a third of people with intrinsic asthma suffer from sinusitis and nasal polyps. Discuss the best treatment with your doctor.

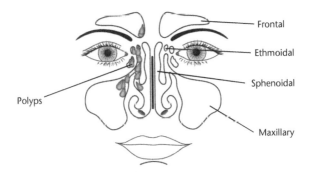

Figure 4(a) The sinuses and polyps – front view

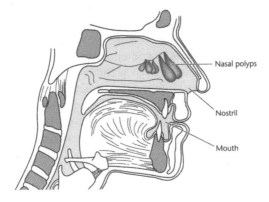

Figure 4(b) The sinuses and polyps – side view

Heartburn

Heartburn (dyspepsia) can arise from several causes, ranging from overindulgence to potentially fatal cancers. So, see your GP if you start experiencing unexplained and persistent heartburn, especially if you're aged 55 years or older or experience other symptoms, such as:

• unintentional weight loss

- difficulty swallowing
- vomiting
- signs of anaemia, such as tiredness and lack of energy, shortness of breath, palpitations and looking pale.

Gastro-oesophageal reflux disease (GORD) – when the stomach's acidic contents enter the oesophagus (food pipe) – causes heartburn. Normally, a valve (sphincter) between the stomach and oesophagus prevents 'reflux'. However, certain meals, changes in posture (especially lying down), certain medications (including some drugs used to treat asthma) and stress may weaken the sphincter, allowing reflux.

People with GORD may regurgitate small amounts of stomach acid into their mouths, from where it can seep into their tracheas and lungs. This can cause a bothersome cough and nocturnal symptoms. Treating GORD may relieve some asthma symptoms.

If you feel that GORD is making your symptoms worse, talk to your pharmacist or doctor. (But always let him or her know you have asthma.) Some changes may also help:

- Lose weight, stop smoking and consume less alcohol, coffee, chocolate and fatty foods.
- Raise the head of the bed. (Try propping the head of your bed up on bricks.)
- Avoid eating close to your bedtime. Food stimulates your stomach to produce acid.

Beta-agonists (page 42), anticholinergics (page 43) and theophylline (page 40) alleviate asthma by relaxing muscle surrounding the airways. But they also relax the sphincter, allowing reflux. Steroid tablets can cause indigestion and ulcers. So, if lifestyle measures don't help, talk to your GP.

Indoor and outdoor pollution

Public Health England estimates that long-term exposure to air pollution directly caused about 29,000 early deaths in the UK during 2008: more than twice the annual death toll from breast cancer. Air pollution potentially contributed to another 200,000 deaths. Indeed, air pollution can lead to serious conditions such as heart disease and cancer, impair lung development and exacerbate COPD and asthma. For example:

- People in towns and cities seem to be more likely to develop asthma due to pollen than those in the country, partly because pollution enhances pollen's ability to trigger immune reactions.
- People with asthma could experience discomfort or symptoms when air pollution is high (listen to the weather forecast). So, spend less time outdoors and don't exercise in front of an open window.
- Pollution levels are much higher in other parts of the world than in the UK; it might be worth checking the air quality of any city you plan to visit.

With cars and lorries belching out toxic fumes, it's easy to forget that, as most of us spend far more time indoors than outside, our exposure to indoor pollution is greater. Sources of indoor pollution include:

- Tobacco smoke – even passive smoking: people with asthma who smoke regularly tend to endure more severe symptoms, have a worse quality of life, make more trips to A&E departments and are more likely to need hospitalization than asthmatics who do not smoke. Smoking also accelerates the decline in lung function. Some people find that second-hand vapour from e-cigarettes irritates their lungs.
- Gas cookers and kerosene heaters may produce nitrogen dioxide.

- Open fires and paraffin may release sulphur dioxide and particulate pollutants.
- Cooking can release particulate matter and aerosols. Stir-frying, for example, creates large amounts of particulate matter.
- Some DIY products, cleaning products, air fresheners, paints, electrical goods and so on may release chemicals that irritate the respiratory tract.

Weather

Weather can affect the risk of suffering asthma and other allergies in several ways. We've seen that cold air can trigger asthma and ozone levels rise on sunny days, while weather patterns influence pollen levels. For example:

- Most flowers release pollen in the early morning, often triggered by changes in humidity.
- Rain can remove pollen from the air.
- Thunderstorms concentrate pollen at ground level. Certain people with hay fever who do not normally experience respiratory symptoms suffer full-blown asthma attacks during some thunderstorms.

If you think a particular weather pattern exacerbates your symptoms, try to limit your exposure.

Poor adherence

The most effective drug is useless unless you take it correctly. Yet 30 to 70 per cent of people with asthma admit poor adherence: they don't take their treatment as suggested by their doctor or asthma nurse. Some deliberately don't follow the advice: they may deny that they are ill, have low expectations of treatment, suffer from psychiatric problems or fail to appreciate the risks, for instance. Others are worried about side effects or find treatment disrupts their lifestyle unacceptably. If this sounds like you, have an open and honest discussion with your GP or asthma nurse.

Often poor adherence is unintentional. People may misunderstand instructions, become confused – especially if they need to take several drugs – or simply forget. Ask your doctor to check that you really need all the drugs. You could keep your steroid by your bedside if you take your anti-inflammatory twice a day. (Obviously, keep medicines out of the reach of children.)

People with physical disabilities may experience difficulties opening packaging or using medication. Pharmacists can suggest alternative packaging or dosing forms, such as avoiding 'child-resistant' pill bottles or using liquid formulations. If you can't use the inhaler correctly, changing the inhaler or using an aid may help.

Some people take excessive amounts of steroid or bronchodilator, usually through fear that they'll suffer a serious attack. A self-management plan helps put you back in control and allows you to increase the dose of medication when your symptoms or peak flow, which measures your lung function (page 26), worsen.

Menstrual cycles and the menopause

Many women find that their asthma symptoms worsen just before their period, probably due to changing hormone levels. Try keeping a diary recording your peak flow and discuss any asthmatic and menstrual symptoms with your doctor or asthma nurse.

Some women develop asthma for the first time after menopause, especially if they are overweight. Some forms of hormone replacement therapy (HRT) may trigger asthma. If you feel that you need HRT, discuss the potential impact on your asthma with your GP. In some cases, there may be an alternative.

3

Diagnosing asthma

Symptoms such as breathlessness, chest pain and cough are not always a reliable way to diagnose and monitor asthma. Indeed, symptoms correlate poorly with lung function and the severity of the underlying inflammation. For instance:

- Some people with severe asthma report fewer and less intense symptoms than people with milder asthma.
- At any given severity, older people typically feel that their symptoms and exacerbations are more severe than younger people.
- Older people are typically less able to perceive bronchoconstriction (narrowing of the airways) following exposure to chemicals than younger asthmatics. So, older people may not appreciate the seriousness of the attack.
- Older people may regard limitations to their activity as inevitable (because of their asthma, age or both) and not a marker of poor control.
- Asthma's symptoms overlap with those of other diseases common in older people.

Lung function tests

Doctors use lung function tests to diagnose asthma, monitor response to treatment and warn of impending attacks. In healthy people, lung function increases until early adolescence and then remains stable until the mid-30s, before declining. So, doctors usually express results of lung function tests as a percentage of those predicted for other people of the same age, sex and height. Doctors generally regard normal lung function as being within 85 per cent of the predicted average value.

Peak flow

Peak flow measures the maximum rate at which air moves when you exhale. This indirectly indicates the airway's diameter. You exhale for a second or two, which doctors convert to litres per minute.

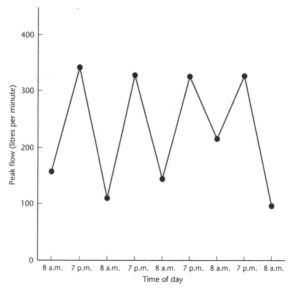

Figure 5 Example of a 'saw-tooth' pattern in severe asthma

An improvement of 60 litres a minute (l/min) or at least 20 per cent after taking a short-acting broncho-dilator (page 42) strongly suggests you have asthma. Your doctor or nurse may ask you to measure peak flow in the morning and evening (sometimes more frequently) for, usually, a couple of weeks. Asthma patients tend to show a greater variation over a day than healthy people and those with some other diseases (Figure 5).

In general, asthma symptoms do not emerge until peak flow declines by 25 per cent or more from your personal best. So, regularly measuring peak flow can warn of an impending exacerbation. In general, peak flow a third or more below your best may suggest poor control. An increase in the normal variation between the peak and the trough may also indicate poor control, increased severity or both. Noting what you were doing when symptoms emerge can help you identify a cause. If your symptoms get worse when vacuuming or making beds, you could be allergic to house dust mites or dander, for example.

Spirometry

Spirometry measures the volume of air expelled in one breath, when you breathe out as hard as you can after breathing in as deeply as possible. This allows doctors to calculate:

- *Forced vital capacity (FVC)* This is the total volume of air expelled forcefully until no more air can be breathed out. In healthy people, FVC is around 60 per cent of lung capacity.
- *Forced expiratory volume in one second (FEV$_1$)* As you breathe out, the volume of air exhaled increases rapidly and then levels off. Healthy people typically

take around four seconds to expel a full breath and usually expel at least 75 per cent of the breath in the first second (FEV$_1$; Figure 6).

Doctors calculate the ratio between FEV$_1$ and FVC. People with asthma have narrow airways, so they exhale more slowly and FEV$_1$ declines. FVC also declines, but less than FEV$_1$. An FEV$_1$:FVC ratio of 75 per cent or less of predicted is a more sensitive indicator of airway obstruction, depends less on the person's effort and is more reproducible than peak flow. Indeed, the ratio may decline (indicating obstruction) when FEV$_1$ is normal.

Normal spirometry while you experience symptoms means that it's unlikely you have asthma. On the other hand, spirometry may be normal when you don't have symptoms. So, you may have to undergo repeated measurements.

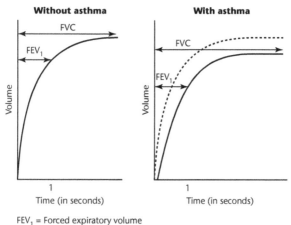

FEV$_1$ = Forced expiratory volume
FVC = Forced vital capacity

Figure 6 FEV$_1$ and FVC in people with and without asthma

Challenge tests

As we've seen, asthmatic airways often constrict when exposed to non-specific triggers such as cold air, dust and tobacco smoke. Doctors use this 'bronchial hyper-reactivity' to help diagnose asthma. For example, a chemical called methacholine constricts airways. The doctor gradually increases the dose of methacholine until FEV_1 declines by 20 per cent. Around 95 per cent of asthmatics need a much lower dose of methacholine to constrict bronchi by 20 per cent than people with healthy lungs.

Other challenge (sometimes called provocation) tests use cold air, saline (a salt solution), exercise, other chemicals (usually histamine or adenosine) or a suspected occupational trigger. Challenge tests may trigger an exacerbation and, as a result, are performed in specialized centres. A challenge test isn't necessarily definitive. Some people with healthy lungs, smokers and those with some other lung diseases show abnormal challenge tests, for instance.

Immune tests

Doctors may suggest tests that determine whether your immune system is over-sensitive to a particular allergen. But if you test positive, the allergen may not be responsible. The immune reaction might not be sufficiently severe to trigger asthma.

During a skin prick test, a fine needle presses a small amount of the suspected allergen into your skin on the inside of your forearm. (I've had this done. It doesn't hurt.) A swelling (weal) surrounded by a red flare 15 minutes or so later suggests you're sensitive to that allergen. The test also includes the fluid used to suspend the allergen (the vehicle), which shouldn't cause symptoms, and histamine to deliberately provoke weal and flare and show the test is working correctly.

Another investigation measures blood levels of an antibody (a protein involved in immune responses) called IgE. A high level suggests that an allergy may underlie your asthma. Again, a positive test is much more common than symptoms caused by the abnormal immune response.

4

Treating asthma in adults

The wide choice of drugs and devices now available for asthma means that you and your doctor or nurse can probably find the right combination of a bronchodilator ('reliever') and an anti-inflammatory ('preventer') to:

- minimize symptoms, including nocturnal and exercise-induced symptoms;
- prevent exacerbations, therefore minimizing your need to use 'rescue' bronchodilators to alleviate asthma attacks;
- achieve the best possible lung function (ideally within 80 per cent of your best or predicted value);
- minimize side effects.

You should agree individual goals for your treatment. Doctors or nurses may focus more on symptoms and lung function, while you may want to spend more time in the garden, return to work or exercise. You can adapt treatment to meet your goals. You may need more intensive therapy if you are planning to run a marathon than if you want to want to play with your kids or grandchildren in the park, for example.

Once you've agreed your goals watch for any signs of poor control. For example, if you can answer yes to one or more of the following questions, you may have poorly controlled asthma and should see your doctor or nurse:

- Have you experienced difficulties sleeping because of asthma, including cough?
- Have new asthma symptoms (cough, wheeze, chest tightness or breathlessness) emerged?
- Have your usual symptoms become more severe during the day?
- Has asthma interfered with your usual activities around the home, at work or college?
- Are you using more than 10 or 12 puffs of bronchodilator a day – around two canisters a month?

The principles of treatment

Asthma management takes, broadly, a two-pronged approach:

- Inhaled corticosteroids and other anti-inflammatory drugs suppress the underlying inflammation. Steroids dampen inflammation too slowly to relieve attacks rapidly.
- Bronchodilators open constricted airways and alleviate exacerbations but don't reduce inflammation.

Your doctor or asthma nurse will adjust the dose and combination of anti-inflammatory drugs and bronchodilators to control your symptoms and optimize lung function following the stepped approach laid out in the *British Guideline on the Management of Asthma* (see <https://www.brit-thoracic.org.uk/guidelines-and-quality-standards/asthma-guideline/>).

You start treatment at the level most likely to minimize symptoms and normalize lung function, then move up to the next step if your asthma remains inadequately controlled. Once your asthma is well controlled for several months, treatment moves down a step. On the other hand, if asthma worsens, treatment can move up a step.

> ### *Travelling with asthma*
>
> Review your action plan and treatment before you travel, so you know when to increase your inhaled steroid dose or start oral steroids. Make sure you have:
>
> - spare preventers and relievers (carry these in your hand luggage);
> - a short course of oral steroids (discuss taking these with you, even if you don't usually have them, with your doctor or nurse);
> - adequate health insurance;
> - information about local emergency and other health services in your destination;
> - discussed travel vaccinations.

Self-management programmes and action plans

Self-management programmes and action plans use these principles individualized to you and your circumstances. Some people want as much control over their treatment as possible and monitor symptoms and peak flow rigorously. Other people would rather take less responsibility. So, be honest with your medical team about how much responsibility you want so they can develop programmes and plans that meet your needs.

Most self-management programmes allow you to recognize declining control based on symptoms, peak flow or both, such as when to:

- seek emergency help;

- increase the dose of inhaled steroids;
- start oral steroids. You may receive an emergency course of steroid tablets.

Anti-inflammatory drugs

Even when you're symptom-free, your lungs probably remain inflamed, increasing the risk of an exacerbation. So, take your anti-inflammatory even when you feel your asthma's well controlled.

Steroids

Steroids are a large group of natural and synthetic chemicals, with a wide range of effects. Corticosteroids are, for instance, different from the 'anabolic' steroids abused by some weight-lifters, athletes and body-builders. You won't start putting on muscle if you take corticosteroids for asthma.

Regularly using inhaled corticosteroids (such as beclomethasone – also called beclometasone – budesonide or fluticasone):

- alleviates asthma symptoms;
- reduces the risk of exacerbations;
- improves lung function;
- enhances quality of life.

You'll use a dose that controls your asthma. The risk of side effects rises as the dose increases, so you should use the lowest dose of inhaled steroid that ensures you meet your treatment goals. If you're worried you're taking too much, speak to your doctor or nurse before cutting back.

Side effects

Inhaled steroids are, generally, relatively safe and less hazardous than poorly controlled asthma. But they can cause side effects, including:

- Inhaled steroids can suppress the mouth's immune defences. So, up to one person in 20 taking inhaled corticosteroids will develop oral candidiasis (thrush in the mouth): white patches around the gums, palates and tongue. Rinsing and spitting after inhaling the steroid or using a spacer (page 46) reduces the risk.
- Between 2 and 6 per cent of people taking inhaled steroids (especially higher doses) develop dysphonia (voice changes).
- Steroids can 'thin the skin' and produce red or purple discolorations, called purpura, caused by blood vessels leaking near the skin's surface. So, you may bruise easily, especially if you're older, taking higher doses or using steroids long term.
- Steroids – again especially high doses and long courses – can a trigger a sudden outbreak of acne in adults, especially on the trunk.
- Steroids taken at high doses, long term, can cause fine downy hair to appear on the sides of the face, upper lip and chin (hirsutism).
- Inhaled steroids, especially at high doses, may increase the risk of diabetes.
- Other serious side effects – including weak bones, cataracts (page 38) and glaucoma (page 38) – occur in less than 1 per cent of people using inhaled steroids. They generally emerge at higher doses, during prolonged treatment or both.

So discuss the risks and benefits with your doctor or asthma nurse. If you don't meet the treatment goals or experience an exacerbation, your GP or asthma nurse might suggest increasing your dose of steroid or adding another drug, after checking that:

- you have taken your existing drugs as prescribed;
- your inhaler technique is good;
- as far as possible, you have eliminated or treated trigger factors, such as smoking, allergens and hay fever;
- the diagnosis is correct;
- you haven't developed another disease that reduces treatment effectiveness.

Oral steroids

You may take steroid tablets, usually prednisolone, generally for a week or two if:

- your asthma remains difficult to control on inhaled steroids;
- you suffer a severe exacerbation;
- you show a potentially dangerous decline in lung function.

Oral steroids deliver a higher dose than their inhaled counterparts. So, oral steroids are highly effective at controlling asthmatic inflammation and can be life-savers. On the other hand, the risk of developing side effects is much greater.

Some side effects emerge soon after you start taking oral steroids, such as mood changes (like feeling anxious, irritable, depressed or 'high') and stomach problems. Others – such as weakness or a rounder face – develop after you've taken oral steroids for several weeks or months, or have received several courses. Elderly asthmatics may be especially prone to these side effects, as they often break down steroids less rapidly than younger people.

People taking steroid tablets long term (for example, for more than three months) or frequently (such as three to four or more times a year) are at risk of potentially serious side effects. So, doctors or nurses should regularly check:

- blood pressure and cholesterol levels, to monitor the risk of heart disease;
- levels of sugar in urine or blood, to check for diabetes;
- bone mineral density, to watch for osteoporosis (brittle bone disease);
- eyes, for cataracts.

We discussed some side effects that can arise with oral steroids (such as skin thinning, acne and hirsutism) when we looked at inhaled steroids. Other side effects of oral steroids include:

- *Withdrawal reactions* Your body can adapt to oral steroids. So, stopping long-term treatment abruptly can trigger, for example, muscle and joint pain, conjunctivitis (red, inflamed eyes), fever, weight loss, runny nose and painful, itchy skin lumps. Always seek advice from a doctor or asthma nurse before stopping or reducing the dose.
- *Chicken pox complications* If you have never suffered chicken pox or shingles, stay away from people with these infections. Oral steroids suppress the immune response. So, the virus responsible for chicken pox and shingles can cause serious complications and even prove fatal in people taking oral steroids. See your GP immediately if you encounter anyone suffering from chicken pox or shingles and are taking oral steroids.
- *Osteoporosis* (exacerbating the age-related decline

in skeletal strength), muscle wasting and weakness, and unusual tiredness. These changes may increase the risk of a fall and, therefore, the risk that you will break a bone. Protect your skeleton with exercise, calcium and vitamin D (ask your doctor, nurse or pharmacist for the amount you need). Doctors can prescribe medicines for osteoporosis.

- *Cataracts* These are cloudy patches in the transparent lens at the front of your eye that focuses light on the retina that lines the back of your eyeball. So, your vision may become blurred or cloudy. Cataracts can cause blindness.

- *Glaucoma*, a build-up of pressure in the eye that can damage the retina. If untreated, glaucoma can damage the nerves that carry signals from the retina to the brain, leading to loss of vision. Eye tests can detect diseases such as glaucoma and cataracts before they affect your vision.

- *Altered production of hormones* Oral steroids can change the balance of hormones in the body. This can increase the amount of fat in the face and shoulders – known as 'moon face' and 'buffalo hump' respectively. Women taking oral steroids may find their periods become irregular or stop.

While these side effects are unpleasant, oral steroids could save your life. Taking your inhaled treatment as recommended, monitoring your symptoms and lung function, and tackling any trigger factors should reduce the likelihood that you'll need oral steroids. But if and when you do need oral steroids, take them as prescribed. You might want to discuss the risks and benefits with your doctor or asthma nurse before you need to resort to the tablets.

Sodium cromoglicate and nedocromil

Sodium cromoglicate (also spelt cromoglycate) and nedocromil stabilize mast cells, a type of blood cell that drives asthma inflammation. However, as they work on only a single type of cell, sodium cromoglicate and nedocromil are generally less effective than inhaled steroids, which have a wider action. Nevertheless, sodium cromoglicate and nedocromil can be valuable for people who cannot or will not take inhaled steroids or for some cases of exercise-induced asthma.

Leukotriene receptor antagonists

Leukotrienes, a group of chemical messengers, constrict the airways, increase secretion of bronchial mucus (which blocks the airways) and drive inflammation. Leukotriene receptor antagonists (such as montelu-kast and zafirlukast) block these messengers and so control asthmatic inflammation. Certain people seem to benefit particularly from leukotriene receptor antag-onists, including those:

- with marked inflammation in their upper airways (for example, allergic rhinitis or nasal polyps);
- with aspirin-sensitive asthma;
- who experience marked bronchoconstriction when they exercise;
- who experience problems using inhalers – montelu-kast and zafirlukast are tablets.

Doctors and nurses can't predict with certainty who will benefit more from adding a leukotriene receptor antagonist rather than a long-acting beta-agonist (page 42) to the steroid. So, if symptoms haven't improved after four and six weeks, it's worth discussing an alternative.

Theophylline

Theophylline, a tablet, is a bronchodilator, loosens bronchial mucus and inhibits a type of white blood cell involved in allergic asthma. Theophylline is, however, a less potent anti-inflammatory than inhaled steroids.

A relatively small difference separates the dose of theophylline that alleviates asthma from that causing side effects, such as abdominal pain, diarrhoea, headache, rapid heartbeat, palpitations, abnormal heart rhythm, insomnia, nausea, nervousness, tremor, vomiting and liver disease. In some patients, the beneficial and 'toxic' doses overlap, and older people seem to be particularly sensitive to theophylline's side effects.

So, the dose needs to be carefully tailored for each person, which may mean regular blood tests, especially as several factors can influence the way the body breaks down theophylline. For instance:

- Smoking and heavy alcohol use can lower levels, reducing theophylline's efficacy.
- Viral infections, heart failure and liver disease can increase levels, potentially causing side effects.
- Numerous drugs that you may take for another condition can influence theophylline levels.

So, tell your doctor and pharmacist:

- you're taking theophylline when you are prescribed a new drug or buying a medicine;
- if you are using herbal medicines or another complementary therapy, some of which can interact with theophylline;
- if the drugs look different. Different brands may release slightly different doses of theophylline. Check that the pharmacist gives you the exact

brand that you have been prescribed. You should change brand only after discussing the switch with your doctor or asthma nurse.

These issues mean that doctors tend to use theophylline only when long-acting beta-agonists and leukotriene receptor antagonists have failed to adequately control symptoms.

Other options

Omalizumab prevents the release of inflammatory mediators triggered by the allergen. Omalizumab is added to the current treatment of adults and adolescents (12 years and older) with unstable severe asthma despite optimized standard therapy.

As a last resort, specialists may try a short course of potent immunosuppressants, such as methotrexate, ciclosporin (also spelt cyclosporine) and oral gold. These drugs are more commonly used to treat other conditions such as rheumatoid arthritis or for preventing the body from rejecting transplanted organs. Immunosuppressants have potentially serious side effects and few patients need to take these drugs of last resort.

Bronchodilators

Bronchodilators relax the ring of muscle surrounding the airways, opening the airway. Two types are used to treat asthma:

- Short-acting bronchodilators ('relievers') ease breathlessness during asthma attacks and prevent exercise-induced symptoms.
- Long-acting bronchodilators (also called long-acting

beta-agonists) are added to anti-inflammatory drugs if you don't meet your treatment goals with inhaled steroids alone.

Short-acting bronchodilators

The bronchial widening produced by short acting beta-agonists peaks within 15 minutes and lasts between four and six hours. So, short-acting beta-agonists alleviate asthma attacks and prevent exercise-induced exacerbations. As asthma attacks can be unpredictable, always carry your bronchodilator with you.

Overusing your bronchodilator may disguise the severity of the underlying disease. It's a bit like papering over the cracks. Using two or more canisters of beta-agonists per month, or more than 10–12 puffs per day, may suggest that your asthma is poorly controlled. Ask your doctor or asthma nurse to review your treatment.

Few people develop side effects – which include tremor, palpitations and muscle cramps – unless they use high doses of bronchodilator. If you feel that your short-acting inhaler is producing side effects, speak to your asthma nurse or GP. Side effects may suggest that you're using too much beta-agonist and you need to change the dose of anti-inflammatory.

Long-acting beta$_2$-agonists

Taken twice daily, long-acting beta$_2$-agonists (LABAs) keep the bronchi open throughout the day and night.

The *British Guideline on the Management of Asthma* suggests using LABAs only when inhaled steroids alone do not adequately control symptoms. So, ensure that you use a combination inhaler containing both a LABA and an inhaled steroid.

Oral beta-agonists

You can take beta-agonists as tablets, capsules or syrups. The tablets slowly release the beta-agonist, producing sustained bronchodilation. Short-acting oral formulations offer a 'reliever' for people unable to use an inhaler. Oral beta-agonists often produce more side effects than their inhaled counterparts.

Anticholinergics

Anticholinergics (also called antimuscarinics) open the airways through a different mechanism from beta-agonists. Traditionally, doctors prescribed anticholinergics for COPD rather than asthma – although between 10 and 15 per cent of patients have both conditions. However, tiotropium is a maintenance bronchodilator (i.e. not for exacerbations) for adults who experienced one or more severe asthma exacerbations in the previous year despite receiving inhaled steroids and LABAs.

Stepping down treatment

Your doctor or nurse will increase the dose and number of drugs until your symptoms are well controlled. However, symptoms usually wax and wane – if, for example, exposure to the allergen changes or your fitness level improves. Furthermore, once the underlying inflammation is well controlled, you need lower doses of steroid to keep your asthma at bay.

So, you should step down therapy once asthma has been well controlled for a reasonable time. Speak to your doctor or asthma nurse if you feel it's time to step down.

Inhaler devices

Unfortunately, many people experience problems using asthma inhalers properly. For instance, poor coordination between actuation (pressing the canister) and inhalation using metered dose inhalers (MDIs) reduces the amount of drug deposited in the lung from about 23 to 7 per cent. Such problems are common: 28 to 68 per cent do not use their MDI or dry powder inhaler (DPI) sufficiently well to benefit from the drug.

To complicate matters further, different inhalers have different techniques. Always read the materials in the pack carefully and ask your doctor or nurse to demonstrate. You should also check your technique with a doctor or nurse if you are considering stepping up treatment.

Metered dose inhalers (MDIs)

MDIs are the most widely used inhaler. Basically,

- press on the canister that contains the drug ('actuation') while breathing in slowly and steadily;
- continue to breathe in after the inhaler has delivered the drug;
- hold your breath for ten seconds.

While many people can use MDIs, some people find timing the inhalation and actuation difficult. Furthermore, some propellant remains in the MDI canister after you have used the drug. So, it can also be difficult to know when you need to replace your inhaler. You could check the insert for the number of doses, then divide by the number of puffs each day; or ask your GP, asthma nurse or pharmacist when to ask for a repeat prescription.

Only between 10 and 20 per cent of the dose of drug inhaled from an MDI reaches the lower airways. Much of the rest deposits in the mouth and throat and is swallowed. You absorb only a tiny amount of the drug you swallow. Nevertheless, even this small amount can cause side effects, especially if you take large doses.

Breath-actuated inhalers and dry powder inhalers (DPIs)

People who have trouble using an MDI may find alternative devices easier. For instance, breath-actuated inhalers do away with the need to coordinate actuation and inhalation. The valve on the inhaler opens only when you inhale. Breathe in slowly and deeply, and hold your breath after the device delivers the drug.

DPIs use the force of the airflow as you inhale to release the drug. So, you don't need to coordinate actuation and inspiration. However, some DPIs need you to breathe in with more force than with an MDI. Some (but not all) DPIs need manual dexterity to use, making them less suitable for some elderly people and other adults with weaknesses due to nerve or muscle

Physical problems using inhalers

Some people with arthritis in their hands or who have difficulty holding certain inhalers find that devices called the Haleraid or Turboaid help. The Haleraid fits on to certain MDIs and allows you to apply pressure with the palm of your hand to activate the canister. The Turboaid fits on to the breath-actuated Turbohalers. Ask your doctor, pharmacist or asthma nurse.

problems, or suffering from arthritis and other physical impairments. Some inhalers include a counter or let you see when you're reaching the end of the drug supply.

Spacers

Spacers increase the amount of drug that reaches the airways, which makes MDIs easier to use, improves effectiveness and reduces side effects. For example:

- Large-volume spacers roughly double the amount of steroid that reaches the lower airway compared to an MDI used alone. So, you may be able to use a lower dose of steroid.
- Spacers reduce the amount of steroid deposited in the back of the mouth and throat, which reduces the risk of dysphonia (page 35) and oral candidiasis (page 35).
- Spacers can help reduce the need to coordinate actuation and inhalation.

You place the MDI in the spacer and breathe through the mouthpiece. A one-way valve closes when you exhale. The distance results in a plume of fine particles and makes coordinating actuation and inhalation easier. During an attack, for example, you actuate a single puff into the spacer then inhale each dose for five breaths, before another actuation. Clean the spacer monthly in detergent and ask your doctor or asthma nurse for a replacement every year.

Nebulizers

Nebulizers use oxygen or compressed air to deliver high doses of bronchodilator during an asthma attack. Some people keep nebulizers at home if, for example, they suffer regular serious exacerbations. You still need to take your anti-inflammatory regularly, and don't delay seeking urgent medical advice during severe acute attacks. Nebulizers can also deliver steroids. However, properly used DPIs and MDIs used with a spacer deliver a greater proportion of the drug into the airway than nebulizers. As a result, nebulizers tend to be used to deliver steroids only if people can't use conventional inhalers.

5

Beyond drugs

Drugs are the mainstay of asthma management. But taking your preventer and using your reliever as required aren't the only ways to improve asthma control. For example, try to do your best to avoid your particular asthma triggers. But avoiding some triggers is easier said than done.

Pollen

Pollen levels vary depending on the time of year and the weather. For example:

- Concentrations of grass pollen usually peak in June and July but can, depending on the climate, peak from May to August.
- Birch pollen levels usually peak in April.
- Nettle tends to release pollen between June and September.

If you are sensitive to a particular pollen, try to reduce your exposure when levels are likely to be highest:

- Stay indoors as far as possible, particularly in the early evening, when the weather forecast announces the pollen count is likely to be high. On any given day, levels are likely to be higher at certain times. Grass pollen counts tend to peak in the morning and late afternoon of warm, dry days with a gentle wind, for example.

- Keep windows at home and in cars closed. Some cars have special filters that reduce the influx of pollen.
- Pollen is sticky. Wash your hair regularly and change clothes after being outside. Wash or wipe any pets that have been outside.
- Get someone else to cut the grass.
- Take holidays by the sea. Pollen counts tend to be lower on the coast than inland.
- Stock your home and garden with plants that produce relatively low levels of pollen, such as hibiscus, periwinkles, azaleas and roses.

House dust mite

Even thorough hoovering with modern vacuum cleaners won't eradicate house dust mites. Mites breed rapidly so numbers return to the previous levels within about a week.

- Beds are often the most important site of mite exposure. Many people with allergies encase their mattress, duvet and pillow in protective covers.
- Wash bedding regularly above 60°C. Colder water washes away the allergen but does not kill the mite.
- Put soft toys in the freezer or wash them in hot water every 14 days.
- Turn the central heating down and open windows.
- Consider decorating with wooden flooring and blinds, which are easier to wash than carpets and thick curtains. If you really want a carpet, buy one with a very short pile.
- When you buy new furniture, consider leather or another surface that's easy to clean.
- Avoid clutter, which can become dusty and is often difficult to clean. Keep books and knick-knacks in

boxes rather than on shelves, and store your belongings in cupboards.

- Vacuum cleaning can shift the allergen from the floor to the air. Using double-walled bags and cleaners fitted with high-efficiency particulate air (HEPA) filtration or electrostatic filters may reduce the amount of dust. If possible ask someone else to vacuum, or wear a mask. Try not to re-enter a room for at least three hours after dusting or vacuuming to allow airborne dust to resettle.
- Some people find asthma symptoms improve after using miticides, which kill the mites. Follow the instructions carefully: some miticides can irritate skin.
- Remove sheepskins, which seem to harbour particularly large mite populations.

Pet dander

Understandably, many people with asthma don't want to re-home their pets. So, try the following to reduce levels of dander:

- Wash bed linen at 60°C or above.
- Wash soft toys at least once a fortnight.
- Keep pets off beds and other soft furnishings.
- Avoid feather pillows. Many people allergic to animal dander cross-react to feathers.
- Ask someone who is not allergic to wash and comb your pet. If you must groom the pet, wear a mask and gloves.
- People allergic to dander and other animals should remember that pet owners and others who work with animals might transport dander on their clothing.

Fungi

Fungi inside and outside the house can trigger asthma in sensitive people. So:

- Regularly wipe mould from bathrooms and windows with cleaners containing an antifungal or a 5 per cent bleach solution. (Wear a mask and gloves.) Clean shower curtains, tiles, shower stall, bath tub and toilet tank. Don't carpet the bathroom.
- Wash walls with an antifungal before decorating. Use paints that contain an antifungal.
- Keep rooms dry and well ventilated. Use a fan or open the window to reduce mould while bathing or cooking. Dry all clothing immediately after washing.
- HEPA filtration and air conditioning may reduce the amount of fungal spores.
- Convection heaters reduce the viability of mould spores and inhibit mildew's spread.
- Bark often contains high levels of mould. If you use a fireplace or wood-burning stove, don't store any firewood inside (or, if there is no alternative, only a day's supply).
- Avoid foam rubber pillows and mattresses, which may be more likely to attract mould than other types of bedding.
- Wardrobes often attract mould. Dry shoes and boots thoroughly before storing. Try a chemical moisture-remover inside wardrobes.
- Empty the waste bin frequently. Keep the bins clean to prevent mould.
- Empty the drip pan under your refrigerator regularly. The combination of food particles and standing water is an ideal breeding ground for mould.

Quit smoking

Smoking (even second-hand) exacerbates asthma and makes the disease more difficult to control. However, fewer than 1 in every 30 smokers manages to quit each year, and more than half relapse within a year. Cutting back seems to increase the likelihood that you'll eventually quit. But you'll probably inhale more deeply to get the same amount of nicotine. So, reduction can take you a large step towards kicking the habit. But don't stop there.

Nicotine's withdrawal symptoms can leave you irritable, restless and anxious as well as experiencing insomnia and craving a cigarette. These withdrawal symptoms generally abate over two weeks or so. Nicotine replacement therapy (NRT) can make life a little easier and seems to increase quit rates.

You can choose from various types of NRT. Patches reduce withdrawal symptoms but have a relatively slow onset of action, while nicotine chewing gum, lozenges, inhalers and nasal spray act more quickly. Talk to your pharmacist, nurse or doctor to find the right NRT for you. If you still find quitting tough even after trying NRT, doctors can prescribe other treatments. But there's no quick fix. You'll still need to be committed to quitting.

Many people have also quit using e-cigarettes. But as these deliver nicotine they remain addictive, and we still don't know if there are any long-term health risks – although they don't deliver the cancer-causing poisons in tobacco. So, again, e-cigarettes can take you a large step towards kicking the habit. But don't stop there.

Tips to help you quit

A few hints may make life easier:

- Set a quit date and keep a diary of problems and situations that tempt you to light up, such as meals, pubs or breaks at work. Find ways to avoid the problem.
- Find something to take your mind off smoking. If you find yourself smoking when you get home in the evening, try a new hobby or exercise.
- Ask your family and friends for advice and support, such as putting up with any bad moods as you quit.
- Keep a note of how much you save and spend at least some of it on yourself.
- Some people find that they become more hungry when they lose weight, so have a healthy snack handy.

Coping with relapses

On some measures, nicotine is more addictive than heroin and cocaine. So try to regard any relapse as a temporary setback. Set yourself another quit date and try again.

It's worth trying to identify why you relapsed:

- Were you stressed out?
- Did you meet up with particular friends?
- Was smoking linked to a particular time, place or event?

Once you know why you slipped you can develop strategies to stop the problem in the future.

Losing weight

Obese and overweight asthmatics typically show greater airway obstruction and are more likely to endure nocturnal symptoms than those who maintain a healthy weight. They're also at increased risk of type 2 diabetes, heart disease and some cancers.

For example, fat within or pressing down on the airway can narrow and change the airway's shape from a circle to a less efficient oval. Abdominal fat may prevent the diaphragm from descending as far as in people of a healthy weight. Losing weight alleviates symptoms and improves diurnal and day-to-day variations in lung function.

Losing excess weight is not easy. However, the following may help:

- Take 30 to 60 minutes of aerobic exercise each day: brisk walking, jogging, taking an aerobics class or using a stationary bike or treadmill will all help you lose weight. You can break the exercise down into chunks of 10 or 15 minutes.
- Keep a food diary or use an app to record everything you eat and drink for a couple of weeks. It's easy to inadvertently pile on extra calories: the odd biscuit, the extra glass of wine or full-fat latte.
- Don't try to lose too much weight too quickly. Steadily losing around a pound or two a week reduces your chance of putting it back on again.
- Set a specific goal, such as losing two stone.
- Set yourself small attainable goals, such as switching from full-fat to skimmed milk, walking 15 minutes during your lunch break each day, going to the gym three times a week, and only indulging in chocolate on Fridays.

- Don't let a slip-up derail your diet. Try to identify why you indulged. Once you know why you slipped you can develop strategies to stop the problem in the future.

If all this fails, try talking to your GP or pharmacist. A growing number of medicines may help kick-start your weight loss, although you'll still need to change your lifestyle.

Psychological factors

It's easy to become caught in a classic vicious circle. Asthma can cause stress, anxiety and depression. In turn, stress, depression and anxiety may worsen asthma. For example:

- Depression can undermine your motivation to follow your doctor's or nurse's advice.
- Asthma, especially if severe or poorly controlled, can cause considerable anxiety. After all, asthma attacks are often frightening and the next attack could be the one that proves fatal. When you're anxious, adrenaline floods into your blood, causing your breathing to become faster. Obviously, changes to respiration worry asthmatics. The adrenaline rush also heightens alertness and the senses, increasing awareness of the changes.
- Anxiety can lead to you becoming over-cautious, so you may needlessly use medication, attend A&E or miss work.
- If you are anxious about side effects, you may not use your inhaler as needed.

So, get help for depression, anxiety and any other psychiatric conditions. The doctor may suggest antidepressants or drugs to alleviate anxiety. Don't dismiss these out of hand. Drugs don't cure the problem but may offer a 'window of opportunity' to improve your asthma control and, in turn, reduce your anxiety or depression.

So, discuss ways to improve your adherence, tackle the triggers or change your self-management plan with your doctor or asthma nurse. Putting yourself in control of your problems is one of the best ways to beat stress, anxiety and depression. On the other hand, feeling that asthma or other problems control you is one of the most common causes of anxiety, depression and stress.

If you need additional help, your GP may be able to recommend a local counsellor. Alternatively, you could contact the British Association for Counselling and Psychotherapy (<www.bacp.co.uk>).

Diet

Studies examining the effect of diet on asthma show mixed results. For example, some studies, but not all, suggest that high levels of salt in the diet increase airway responsiveness and that diets high in oily fish (such as mackerel, fresh tuna and fresh salmon) seem to protect against asthma. While these results are mixed, reducing salt consumption protects against raised blood pressure, while diets high in oily fish seem to reduce the risk of several other conditions, including heart disease. You could cut your salt intake and increase your consumption of fatty fish and see if your symptoms improve.

Certain foods (notably milk, egg and wheat) and, as we've seen, some additives and preservatives (e.g.

tartrazine) may precipitate asthma in sensitive people. However, don't cut milk, eggs and other basic foods from your diet without advice from a dietician. If you feel that foods exacerbate your symptoms, discuss your concerns with your doctor or asthma nurse.

Complementary and alternative medicines

Complementary and alternative medicines (CAMs) are increasingly popular to, for example, open airways, aid relaxation and calm breathing. Nevertheless, many conventional doctors and nurses remain sceptical, partly because few CAMs undergo the same rigorous scrutiny as modern medicines. But clinical studies are expensive and pharmaceutical companies fund most trials, so this isn't surprising.

Cynics add that the placebo effect accounts for most of CAMs' benefits. In other words, if you think that treatment will work, you'll probably feel better. The symptoms and severity of asthma wax and wane, even without treatment. But if you're using a CAM, you might attribute the improvement to the treatment. However, these effects contribute to conventional medicine's benefits.

Cynics may point out that few studies show that CAMs improve lung function in people with asthma. However, improvements in measures of asthma control – such as limitation of activity, shortness of breath and wheezing – are not necessarily linked to changes in lung function. So, a CAM may improve symptoms and enhance quality of life, even if peak flow doesn't change markedly.

Breathing techniques

Some complementary therapies make sense biologically. If a technique improves breathing, it's logical that it might improve asthma. Alexander therapy, for example, corrects bad posture, brings the body into 'natural alignment' and aids relaxation. Bad posture can hinder the chest's movement and compress the airways. Many actors, musicians and singers find that the Alexander technique enhances their ability to project their voice and improves stamina. Some asthma patients find that the Alexander technique improves their symptoms and reduces their need for medicine.

Indeed, before modern drugs, patients and physicians relied on breathing exercises to control asthma. Even today many asthma patients still show poor breathing techniques that could exacerbate symptoms. For instance, people with asthma may breathe through their mouth only, or may not use their chest muscles correctly. Other people with asthma breathe too rapidly (hyperventilation).

Dysfunctional breathing can exacerbate asthma and even trigger attacks. So, learning to breathe correctly can improve asthma and help you relax. For instance, a yogic breath-control exercise called pranayama slightly reduces airway hyper-responsiveness (page 4). Buteyko seems to improve symptoms and reduce bronchodilator use.

Doctors at Papworth Hospital near Cambridge developed a sequence of breathing and relaxation exercises for asthma during the 1960s. When you're stressed or anxious you probably take rapid, shallow breaths using, predominately, the muscles at the top of your chest. The Papworth technique counters 'over-breathing' by encouraging more relaxed breathing using the abdomen and diaphragm. Essentially, patients drop their shoulders, relax their abdomens and breathe deeply and calmly, which seems to reduce the severity of asthma symptoms and alleviate anxiety and depression.

Relaxation

Don't underestimate relaxation. CAMs such as massage, reflexology, hypnosis and so on can help you relax, and this, in turn, will help alleviate stress-related symptoms and improve your quality of life.

Muscle relaxation could conceivably improve lung function in patients with asthma. One review, for example, reported that 9 out of 17 trials examining herbal treatments showed improved lung function. However, determining which herbs work can be difficult: one Chinese herb decoction (*Ding Chuan Tang*), which improved airway hyper-responsiveness in children with stable asthma, contains nine components. More than one plant may be responsible for the benefits, each plant may contain thousands of potentially active ingredients and the plants may interact to enhance effectiveness or reduce side effects.

Despite the benefits offered by CAMs for some people at least, *never* stop taking your conventional medicines and be sceptical if anyone claims to be able to 'cure' asthma or relies on one or two dramatic cases. A common misconception suggests that because CAMs are natural they are safe. However, some herbs, for example, can interfere with other drugs, causing side effects, or contain salicylates and may therefore trigger symptoms in people with aspirin-sensitive asthma. So, if you want to try a CAM, learn as much as you can about the treatment, see a reputable therapist, keep a

diary of symptoms to see if there is any improvement
and inform your GP, nurse or pharmacist.

A final word

This short book briefly introduces asthma's causes and
treatment. I hope it inspires you to learn more from
the full book, Asthma UK (<www.asthma.org.uk>) and
other patient groups or your GP and asthma nurse.
The more you understand, the better you'll be able to
control your asthma.

It's worth making the effort. Better care could
prevent up to 90 per cent of deaths and 75 per cent
of admissions to hospital due to asthma, as well as
enhancing your quality of life, helping you perform
the normal activities of daily life everyone else seems
to take for granted, and reducing the time you take sick
from work. Getting your asthma under control helps
you live life to the full. I wish you well.